Table of Contents

Introduction

The ketogenic diet is a high-fat, adequate-protein, low-carbohydrate diet that in medicine is used mainly to treat hard-to-control (refractory) epilepsy in children. The diet forces the body to burn fats rather than carbohydrates.

Normally carbohydrates in food are converted into glucose, which is then transported around the body and is important in fueling brain function. But if little carbohydrate remains in the diet, the liver converts fat into fatty acids and ketone bodies, the latter passing into the brain and replacing glucose as an energy source. An elevated level of ketone bodies in the blood (a state called ketosis) eventually lowers the frequency of epileptic seizures. Around half of children and young people with epilepsy who have tried some form of this diet saw the number of seizures drop by at least half, and the effect persists after discontinuing the diet. Some evidence shows that adults with epilepsy may benefit from the diet and that a less strict regimen, such as a modified Atkins diet, is similarly effective. Side effects may include constipation, high cholesterol, growth slowing, acidosis, and kidney stones.

The original therapeutic diet for paediatric epilepsy provides just enough protein for body growth and repair, and sufficient calories to maintain the correct weight for age and height. The classic therapeutic ketogenic diet was developed for treatment of paediatric epilepsy in the 1920s and was widely used into the next decade, but its popularity waned with the introduction of effective anticonvulsant medications. This classic ketogenic diet contains a 4:1 ratio by weight of fat to combined protein and carbohydrate. This is achieved by excluding high-carbohydrate foods such as starchy fruits and vegetables, bread, pasta, grains, and sugar, while increasing the consumption of foods high in fat such as nuts, cream, and butter. Most dietary fat is made of molecules called long-chain triglycerides (LCTs). However, medium-chain triglycerides (MCTs)—made from fatty acids with shorter carbon chains than LCTs—are more ketogenic. A variant of the classic diet known as the MCT ketogenic diet uses a form of coconut oil, which is rich in MCTs, to provide around half the calories. As less overall fat is needed in this variant of the diet, a greater proportion of carbohydrate and protein can be consumed, allowing a greater variety of food choices.

In 1994, Hollywood producer Jim Abrahams, whose son's severe epilepsy was effectively controlled by the diet, created the Charlie Foundation for Ketogenic Therapies to further promote diet therapy. Publicity included an appearance on NBC's Dateline program and ...First Do No Harm (1997), a made-for-television film starring Meryl Streep. The foundation sponsored a research study, the results of which—announced in 1996—marked the beginning of renewed scientific interest in the diet.

Possible therapeutic uses for the ketogenic diet have been studied for many additional neurological disorders, some of which include: Alzheimer's disease, amyotrophic lateral sclerosis, headache, neurotrauma, pain, Parkinson's disease, and sleep disorders.

Keto basics

The ketogenic diet is a very low carb, high fat diet that shares many similarities with the Atkins and low carb diets.

It involves drastically reducing carbohydrate intake and replacing it with fat. This reduction in carbs puts your body into a metabolic state called ketosis.

When this happens, your body becomes incredibly efficient at burning fat for energy. It also turns fat into ketones in the liver, which can supply energy for the brain.

Ketogenic diets can cause significant reductions in blood sugar and insulin levels. This, along with the increased ketones, has some health benefits.

The keto diet is a low carb, high fat diet. It lowers blood sugar and insulin levels and shifts the body's metabolism away from carbs and toward fat and ketones.

Different types of ketogenic diets

There are several versions of the ketogenic diet, including:

Standard ketogenic diet (SKD): This is a very low carb, moderate protein and high fat diet. It typically contains 70% fat, 20% protein, and only 10% carbs (9Trusted Source).

Cyclical ketogenic diet (CKD): This diet involves periods of higher carb refeeds, such as 5 ketogenic days followed by 2 high carb days.

Targeted ketogenic diet (TKD): This diet allows you to add carbs around workouts.

High protein ketogenic diet: This is similar to a standard ketogenic diet, but includes more protein. The ratio is often 60% fat, 35% protein, and 5% carbs.

However, only the standard and high protein ketogenic diets have been studied extensively. Cyclical or targeted ketogenic diets are more advanced methods and primarily used by bodybuilders or athletes.

The information in this book mostly applies to the standard ketogenic diet (SKD), although many of the same principles also apply to the other versions.

What is ketosis?

Ketosis is a metabolic state in which your body uses fat for fuel instead of carbs.

It occurs when you significantly reduce your consumption of carbohydrates, limiting your body's supply of glucose (sugar), which is the main source of energy for the cells.

Following a ketogenic diet is the most effective way to enter ketosis. Generally, this involves limiting carb consumption to around 20 to 50 grams per day and filling up on fats, such as meat, fish, eggs, nuts, and healthy oils.

It's also important to moderate your protein consumption. This is because protein can be converted into glucose if consumed in high amounts, which may slow your transition into ketosis.

Practicing intermittent fasting could also help you enter ketosis faster. There are many different forms of intermittent fasting, but the most common method involves limiting food intake to around 8 hours per day and fasting for the remaining 16 hours.

Blood, urine, and breath tests are available, which can help determine whether you've entered ketosis by measuring the amount of ketones produced by your body.

Certain symptoms may also indicate that you've entered ketosis, including increased thirst, dry mouth, frequent urination, and decreased hunger or appetite.

Ketosis is a metabolic state in which your body uses fat for fuel instead of carbs. Modifying your diet and practicing intermittent fasting can help you enter ketosis faster. Certain tests and symptoms can also help determine whether you've entered ketosis.

Ketogenic diets can help you lose weight
A ketogenic diet is an effective way to lose weight and lower risk factors for disease.

In fact, research shows that the ketogenic diet may be as effective for weight loss as a low fat diet.

What's more, the diet is so filling that you can lose weight without counting calories or tracking your food intake.

One review of 13 studies found that following a very low carb, ketogenic diet was slightly more effective for long-term weight loss than a low fat diet. People who followed the keto diet lost an average of 2 pounds (0.9 kg) more than the group that followed a low fat diet.

What's more, it also led to reductions in diastolic blood pressure and triglyceride levels.

Another study in 34 older adults found that those who followed a ketogenic diet for 8 weeks lost nearly five times as much total body fat as those who followed a low fat diet.

The increased ketones, lower blood sugar levels, and improved insulin sensitivity may also play a key role.

Other health benefits of keto
The ketogenic diet actually originated as a tool for treating neurological diseases such as epilepsy.

Studies have now shown that the diet can have benefits for a wide variety of different health conditions:

Heart disease. The ketogenic diet can help improve risk factors like body fat, HDL (good) cholesterol levels, blood pressure, and blood sugar.

Cancer. The diet is currently being explored as an additional treatment for cancer, because it may help slow tumor growth.

Alzheimer's disease. The keto diet may help reduce symptoms of Alzheimer's disease and slow its progression.

Epilepsy. Research has shown that the ketogenic diet can cause significant reductions in seizures in epileptic children.

Parkinson's disease. Although more research is needed, one study found that the diet helped improve symptoms of Parkinson's disease.

Polycystic ovary syndrome. The ketogenic diet can help reduce insulin levels, which may play a key role in polycystic ovary syndrome.

Brain injuries. Some research suggests that the diet could improve outcomes of traumatic brain injuries.

Slow Cooker Crack Chicken

WHAT IS CRACK CHICKEN?

So, basically, crack chicken is kind of a big craze going around right now. You'll find "crack" recipes for pork, pot roast, pasta, and dips.

What all of these "crack" dishes have in common are 3 key ingredients:

Ranch seasoning

Cream cheese

Bacon

That's all, folks. That's the secret, right there. Just those three simple, delicious ingredients will make any meal completely and utterly addictive.

RECIPE INGREDIENTS

So, for this to classify as "crack", we really only need three things: ranch seasoning mix, cream cheese, and bacon. If you're planning to make yourself some "crack" and you've already got those ingredients, the rest is so simple.

Here's what you'll need:

- low sodium chicken broth
- ranch seasoning mix
- chicken breasts
- cream cheese
- cheddar cheese
- bacon

For serving:

- green onions
- fresh parsley

HOW TO MAKE CRACK CHICKEN IN THE SLOW COOKER

1. Prep: Pour chicken broth into your slow cooker and stir in ranch seasoning mix.

Add chicken breasts to the slow cooker and stir around to coat the chicken.

2. Slow Cook: Cover with the lid and set on LOW for 5 to 6 hours or on HIGH for 2 to 3 hours.

3. Shred: When done, remove the lid and shred the chicken in the slow cooker using two forks. Use shredder claws, if you can – it's MUCH easier.

4. Stir In: Stir in your cream cheese and 1 ½ cups shredded cheddar cheese until completely melted and combined.

5. Top: Top your chicken with remaining cheddar cheese and chopped bacon.

6. Serve: Garnish with green onions and parsley.

Slow cooker crack chicken topped with bacon and herbs and being stirred

WHAT IF I DON'T HAVE RANCH SEASONING MIX?

If you don't have ranch seasoning mix, have no fear! You can easily make your own right at home. All you have to do is combine 1/2 teaspoon garlic powder, ½ teaspoon onion powder, ½ teaspoon dried dill weed, ½ teaspoon dried chives, and season with salt and pepper, to taste.

Tadah, now you have your very own ranch seasoning mix.

SERVING IDEAS

I love to serve shredded slow cooker crack chicken on a sandwich. Give it to me on a seeded and toasted bun ALL day and I'll be happy.

Here are some other yummy ways to serve crack chicken:

To top your favorite pasta (or zoodles)

In a wrap or in lettuce cups

Over rice or quinoa (or riced cauliflower)

On top of a baked potato or mashed potatoes

On top of a pizza (I'm thinking like a BBQ chicken pizza but instead Crack chicken pizza!)

Or simply eat it straight up as a dip with tortilla chips or veggies like you would with a Buffalo chicken dip.

HOW TO STORE AND REHEAT LEFTOVERS

You want to make sure you cool your slow cooker crack chicken completely before storing. Then, keep it in an airtight container in your refrigerator for about 3 days.

To reheat, simmer your crack chicken over medium-low heat until heated through. Add chicken broth, if needed to thin it out. Top with some fresh cheddar cheese and green onions.

Keto Crack Chicken in the Crock Pot

This Crack Chicken in the Crock Pot is keto friendly and low carb. But you don't have to follow a low carb lifestyle to enjoy it. The whole family will love this creamy, cheesy chicken dish.

Ingredients

- 1/2 cup chicken broth
- 1 Hidden Valley Ranch seasoning packet
- 2 pounds of defrosted chicken breasts
- 8 oz package of Philadelphia Cream Cheese cut into chunks
- 8 slices cooked and crumbled bacon
- 1/2 cup shredded cheddar cheese

Instructions

1. Add chicken broth to the slow cooker and stir in Hidden Valley Ranch seasoning packet. Then add defrosted chicken breasts.

2. Cover and cook for 4 hours on high or 8 hours on low.

3. After the cook time has ended, shred the chicken with two forks.

4. Add chunks of cut up Philadelphia Cream Cheese, bacon and shredded cheddar. Stir ingredients.

5. Cover the crock pot again, and cook for an additional 5-10 minutes, until the cream cheese has melted.

Keto Chicken Broccoli Casserole with Cauliflower

Ingredients

- 12 oz chopped and cooked chicken breasts

- 12 oz frozen riced cauliflower

- 3 cups broccoli florets, chopped

- 1 tsp garlic powder

- 1 tsp onion powder
- 4 oz cream cheese, softened and cut into small pieces
- 1.5 cups shredded cheddar cheese
- 1/8 tsp pepper
- 1/4 tsp salt

Instructions

1. Preheat oven to 350 degrees. Cook your chicken in a pan and cut into cubes.
2. Microwave the riced cauliflower according to package directions.
3. Pour into a large bowl and added cut broccoli florets.
4. Add cut up pieces of softened cream cheese, garlic and onion powders, and 2 eggs to bowl.
5. Add 1 cup of shredded cheese and cooked chicken to bowl. Add salt and pepper to taste.
6. Mix well to combine all the ingredients.
7. Transfer mixture to a greased 8x8 casserole dish. Top with 1/2 cup shredded cheddar.

8. Bake for 40 minutes at 350 degrees.

Crack Chicken Casserole

This Keto Crack Chicken Casserole is addictive! Cheese and bacon combine with chicken in this creamy low carb dish.

Ingredients

- 2.5 cups Chicken, cooked cubes
- 1 cup bacon, cooked and chopped
- ¼ cup onion, diced
- 1 cup shredded cheddar cheese
- 3 eggs
- 2 tbsp sour cream
- ½ cup heavy cream
- ½ cup ranch dressing

Instructions

1. Preheat oven to 350 degrees.

2. Cook chicken and cut into cubes.

3. Place chicken into the bottom of an 8x8 casserole dish.

4. Sprinkle half of the cooked and chopped bacon on top of the chicken.

5. Sprinkle the diced onion on top of the bacon in the pan.

6. Cover with 1/2 cup of shredded cheese

7. In a medium bowl, mix eggs, cream, sour cream, and ranch dressing.

8. Pour over the chicken and bacon.

9. Top with the remainder of cheese and bacon.

10. Bake for 35 minutes. Cover with foil for the last 10 minutes of cooking time.

11. Remove from oven and let rest for 5 minutes before serving.

Crock Pot Crustless Pizza

This Crock Pot Crustless Pizza is so easy to make and can be made to fit your family's favorites!

Cook Time: 4 hoursTotal Time: 4 hours 10 minutes Servings: 10 servings Calories: 374kcal Author: Aunt Lou

Ingredients

- 2 lbs ground beef
- garlic salt pepper and dried minced onion to taste
- 2 cups shredded mozzarella cheese
- 14 oz jar pizza sauce
- 2 cups shredded pizza blend cheese
- Your favorite pizza toppings

Instructions

1. Brown your beef and seasonings in a skillet on the stove over medium/high heat and drain
2. Put your beef and mozzarella in a bowl and mix it together
3. Spray your crock pot lightly with cooking spray
4. Evenly spread out your beef mixture in your crock pot

5. Pour your pizza sauce across the top and spread out evenly

6. Top with your pizza blend cheese and toppings

7. Cover and cook on low for around 4 hours

Pulled Pork Lettuce Wrap Meal Prep

Ingredients

- 1 pound boneless pork shoulder

- 1/4 tsp Salt

- 1/4 tsp Pepper

- 1 tbs favorite spice seasoning optional

- 1 medium yellow onion chopped

- 1/4 tsp Garlic Powder

- 1 cup chicken broth

- For Serving

- butter lettuce leaves

- Cherry Tomatoes

- mustard

Instructions

1. Combine all ingredients in a 5-quart or larger slow cooker.
2. Cover and cook on HIGH for 6 hours.
3. Allow to cool, then shred with a fork.
4. Store shredded pork in the fridge for up to one week.
5. Serve with butter lettuce leaves, tomato, mustard, and any of your favorite toppings.

Notes

Nutrition for 1 out of 3 servings:

28g Protein | 4g Carbs | 24g Fat | 1g Fiber | 363 Calories

*Nutrition includes lettuce, tomato and mustard.

Slow Cooker Mexican Chicken Soup

Ingredients

- 400 grams boneless skinless chicken breast
- 1 14 oz can Fire-roasted plum tomato (ref note 1)
- 2 tspn oil
- 1 medium onion Finely Chopped
- 1 tbsp Minced garlic
- 1 red bell pepper Chopped
- 1.5 tsp Roasted Cumin powder
- 1 tsp Dried Oregano
- 1.5 tsp Chipotle chilli powder (ref note 2)
- 1 tsp paprika (Optional)
- 1.5 cups chicken stock
- 1 cup half and half
- 1/2 Cup Cream Cheese (room temperature)
- 1 cup cheddar cheese (or Mexican blend)
- Salt to taste
- Fresh Cilantro leaves for garnishing

Instructions

TO MAKE IN SLOW COOKER

1. Take oil in a pan. Once hot, put minced garlic, followed by onion. Fry till Onion starts to soften a little bit and it is aromatic.

2. To a pre-heated Slow cooker, add chicken breast, crushed tomatoes, cooked Onion and garlic mixture, all the spices, warm Chicken Stock and salt.

3. Cover and let it cook on high 3 hours.

4. To the Crock-Pot, stir in chopped bell peppers, Cream, cream cheese, Shredded cheese. Further, cook on high for 20-30 minutes until all the cheese has melted.

5. At the end of cooking using two forks shred the chicken breast.

6. While serving, top it with fresh cilantro, Sour cream, Avocados.

TO MAKE IN AN INSTANT POT

1. Set the Instant Pot to Saute mode. Once hot add oil.

2. Add minced garlic and chopped Onion to the pot. Saute until onion has softened and it is aromatic.

3. Add Cumin powder, Chipotle Chilli Powder, Oregano, Paprika. Saute for 30 seconds. (By sauteing the spices in oil, it develops flavour. This step can be skipped)

4. Stir in Roasted Tomatoes, Chicken Stock. Scarp the bottom of the pot to release any stuck brown bits. Add salt.

5. Add Chicken Breast to the pot. Cover the lid and cook on Manual /High-Pressure mode for 8 minutes.

6. Let the pressure release naturally for 10 minutes followed by Manually releasing the rest of the pressure.

7. Carefully remove Chicken breast in a plate and shred the chicken breast using forks.

8. To the pot, add chopped bell pepper, Softened Cream Cheese, Cheddar Cheese and half & half. Stir well until all the cheese has melted.

9. Add back the shredded chicken to the pot. Stir well.

10. While serving garnish with fresh coriander leaves.

Notes

In case Roasted Tomatoe is not available, Use regular Canned Tomatoes.

Chipotle Powder can be substituted by Smoked paprika.

Sauteing onion and garlic in oil is to caramelize and develope flavours. You can certainly skip it and dump all the ingridents to the slow cooker/Instant pot and cook , followed by adding rest of the ingredients.

I don't like to cook Cheese or cream for a longer time as it kills the delicate flavour. So I always prefer to add dairy towards the end.

You can also use Frozen Chicken Breast if you are making the Soup in an Instant Pot(That's the beauty of Instant Pot). Just reduce the amount of stock to 1 cup. Cook on high for 12 minutes, followed by 10 minutes of Natural pressure release.

Nutrition

Serving: 100g | Calories: 377kcal | Carbohydrates: 11g | Protein: 28g | Fat: 25g | Saturated Fat: 13g | Cholesterol: 120mg | Sodium: 446mg | Potassium: 607mg | Fiber: 1g | Sugar: 4g | Vitamin A: 1939IU | Vitamin C: 34mg | Calcium: 262mg | Iron: 2mg

Slow Cooker Spaghetti Squash And Meatballs

Ingredients

- 1 medium spaghetti squash
- 1 1/2 cups crushed tomatoes
- 1/2 tsp salt
- 1/2 tsp garlic powder
- 1/4 tsp pepper
- 1/4 tsp dried oregano
- 16 gluten-free chicken meatballs such as Al Fresco
- 2 tbsp butter or olive oil
- Additional salt and pepper to taste

Instructions

1. Cut spaghetti squash in half, crosswise. Place in the bottom of a 6 quart slow cooker, cut-side down.
2. In a processor or blender, combine tomatoes, salt, garlic powder, pepper and oregano. Puree until smooth. Pour into bottom of slow cooker.
3. Place meatballs over tomatoes, around spaghetti squash. Cook on low for 6 to 7 hours or on high for 3 to 4 hours.
4. Using tongs and kitchen gloves, remove spaghetti squash from slow cooker. Scoop out seeds and discard. Scoop out flesh into a sieve or colander and let drain a few minutes to reduce moisture. Transfer to a bowl and toss with butter or olive oil.
5. Divide between 4 plates and top with sauce and meatballs.

Recipe Notes

Serves 4. Each serving has 11.8 g of carbs and 1.92 g of fiber. Total NET CARBS = 9.88 g.

Food energy: 235kcal

Total fat: 13.52g

Calories from fat: 121

Cholesterol: 80mg

Carbohydrate: 11.80g

Total dietary fiber: 1.92g

Protein: 15.39g

Sodium: 504mg

Healthy Slow Cooker Chicken Chile Verde

Incredible comforting slow cooker chicken chile verde. Healthy, satisfying and packed with protein. Serve with corn tortillas, avocado, rice and/or beans! Paleo-friendly.

Ingredients

- 2 pounds tomatillos, husked (paper skins, removed) and cut in half
- 4 Poblano or Anaheim peppers
- 2-3 jalapeños, depending on your spice preference
- 6 garlic cloves
- 1 - 4 oz can diced green chiles
- 1 bunch of organic cilantro
- juice of 1 lime
- 2 teaspoons ground cumin
- 2 teaspoons dried oregano
- 1/4 teaspoon salt, plus more to taste
- Freshly ground black pepper
- 3/4 cup low-sodium chicken broth
- 2 pounds Just BARE Boneless Skinless Chicken Thighs
- 1 large yellow onion, diced

Instructions

1. Place tomatillos cut side down, poblano peppers, jalapeños and unpeeled garlic cloves on a foil-lined large baking sheet. If necessary you can use two baking sheets. Place in the oven under the broiler setting for 8-10 minutes or until the tomatillos and peppers begin to roast and blacken. If you don't have broiler in your oven, you can put the oven at 425 degrees F (this option may take longer).

2. Transfer the poblano and jalapeno peppers to a plastic Ziploc bag and zip it tight (leave the tomatillos and garlic on the baking sheet for now). This allows the peppers to steam in the bag and after 5-10 minutes you should be able to remove the skin, stem and seeds off the peppers. It's okay if you don't remove the skin completely -- the most important part is removing the seeds and stems.

3. While the peppers are steaming in the bag, add tomatillos to a blender. You'll notice that they probably got juicy during the roasting. That's okay; you'll want to add all those juices to the blender too! Peel garlic cloves and add them to the blender along

with the peppers, green chiles, cilantro, lime juice, cumin, oregano, salt, pepper and chicken broth. Blend the ingredients until they are well combined.

4. Add chicken thighs and diced onions to slow cooker, pour tomatillo-chile sauce all over the top of the chicken and stir to combine. Cover and cook on high for 3 hours or low for 7 hours.

5. Before serving, remove chicken with a slotted spoon and shred with a fork. Add back to slow cooker and mix in with a spoon. Taste and adjust seasoning as necessary. Serve with brown rice, corn tortilla, tortilla chips, and/or beans. Serves 6.

Nutrition

Servings: 6 servings

Serving size: 1 serving

Calories: 302kcal

Fat: 8.5g

Saturated fat: 1.3g

Carbohydrates: 25.9g

Fiber: 7g

Sugar: 5.5g

Protein: 33.3g

Thai Slow Cooker Zucchini Lasagna

INGREDIENTS

For The Zoodles:

- 4 Large Zucchinis, * Read notes!
- 1 Tbsp Salt
  For The Lasagna:
- 2 Tbsp Coconut oil
- 1 Pound Extra-lean ground turkey (I used 99% fat free)
- 1 Cup Onion, diced
- 1 Tbsp + 2 tsp Fresh garlic, minced
- 1/2 Tbsp Fresh ginger, minced

- Pepper
- 1 Cup Light coconut milk
- 1/4 Cup Natural creamy peanut butter
- 1/4 Cup Reduced sodium soy sauce
- 2 Tbsp Coconut sugar
- 1 Tbsp Rice vinegar
- 1 Tbsp Fresh lime juice
- 1 Tbsp Fish sauce
- 1-2 Tbsp Sriracha
- 15 Oz Light ricotta cheese
- 1 Large Egg
- 1/2 Cup Cilantro, roughly chopped
- 2 Cups Nappa cabbage, roughly chopped
- 1/2 Cup Water chestnuts, diced
- 8 Ounces Mozzarella cheese, grated (about 2 tightly packed cups)
- 1 Large Red pepper, diced
  For Garnish:
- Cilantro, diced
- Green onion, diced

- Roasted peanuts, diced

- Bean sprouts, roughly chopped

INSTRUCTIONS

1. Preheat the oven to 350 degrees.

2. Using a mandolin, slice the zucchini into thin slices, about 1/8 inch thick. Lay them out flat onto 2 cookie sheets and sprinkle with 1 Tbsp salt (it's okay if some zoodles overlap on the pan.

3. Bake them for 15-20 minutes, until just lightly beginning to brown, to get all the moisture out.

4. While the zoodles cook, heat the coconut oil over medium/high heat in the large pan. Add in the ground turkey, diced onion, garlic, ginger and a pinch of pepper. Cook until the onion is soft and the turkey is browned, about 10-12 minutes, making sure to break up the turkey as it cooks.

5. Once cooked, add in the coconut milk, peanut butter, soy sauce, coconut sugar, rice vinegar, lime juice, fish

sauce and 1 Tbsp of the sriracha. Bring to a boil and boil for 3 minutes, stirring very often so the bottom doesn't burn. Then, reduce the heat to medium and simmer until the sauce is thick and creamy and begins to reduce, about 2-4 minutes. Stir occasionally so it doesn't burn. Adjust sriracha to taste. Set aside

6. Once the zoodles are cooked, transfer them to a long piece of paper towel, cover with another piece of paper towel, and gently press out as much excess moisture as you can. Repeat with a fresh layer of paper towel on top. Set aside.

7. In a medium bowl, use a fork to beat together the ricotta cheese, egg and another pinch of pepper. Set aside.

To Layer:

8. Spray the bottom of a 7 quart slow cooker with cooking spray. Spread in half of the turkey mixture evenly. Then, layer half the zucchini noodles in a single layer, lightly overlapping them, followed by

half the ricotta mixture. Gently spread out the ricotta to "seal in" in the zoodles.

9. Sprinkle half the cilantro on, followed by half the cabbage and half the water chestnuts. Finally, sprinkle with half the Mozzarella cheese.

10. Repeat the layers once more, except only use half of the remaining Mozzarella cheese on top. Then, add the diced red pepper on top of the last layer of Mozzarella.

11. Cover your slow cooker and cook on low for 4-5 hours, or until everything is melted and the sides of the lasagna are brown. Sprinkle on the remaining cheese and let stand, covered, until melted.

12. Sprinkle with ALL the garnishes and DEVOUR!

NUTRITION INFO:

Calories: 341kcal (17%) Carbohydrates: 15.5g (5%) Protein: 31.2g (62%) Fat: 17.1g (26%) Saturated Fat: 10.1g (63%) Polyunsaturated Fat: 0.4g Monounsaturated Fat: 1.7g Cholesterol: 76.7mg (26%) Sodium: 1634.1mg (71%)

Potassium: 338.5mg (10%) Fiber: 2.6g (11%) Sugar: 7.6g (8%) Vitamin A: 2055IU (41%) Vitamin C: 45mg (55%) Calcium: 201mg (20%) Iron: 1.2mg (7%)

Low Carb Crock Pot Chicken Fajita Soup

Crock Pot Chicken Fajita Soup is easy to make and tasty. The entire family will enjoy this Low Carb Crock Pot Chicken Fajita Soup recipe. It's also budget friendly.

Course: Soup

Keyword: crock pot chicken fajita soup

Servings: 8

Calories: 171 kcal

Ingredients

- 2 lbs boneless skinless chicken breasts mine were frozen
- 2 cans of diced tomatoes 14.5 oz
- 2 cups chicken broth
- 2 tablespoons taco seasoning I used homemade
- 2 teaspoons minced garlic
- 1/2 cup onion chopped
- 1 green bell pepper chopped
- 1 red bell pepper chopped

Instructions

1. Combine all the ingredients in the crockpot.
2. Cook on low for 6-8 hours.
3. Shred and chop the chicken.
4. Stir to combine the flavors.

Recipe Notes

Serve with tortillas or tortilla chips.

Nutrition Facts

Crock Pot Chicken Fajita Soup

Amount Per Serving

Calories 171 Calories from Fat 36

% Daily Value*

Fat 4g6%

Saturated Fat 1g6%

Cholesterol 73mg24%

Sodium 349mg15%

Potassium 741mg21%

Carbohydrates 8g3%

Fiber 2g8%

Sugar 4g4%

Protein 26g52%

Vitamin A 1144IU23%

Vitamin C 50mg61%

Calcium 42mg4%

Iron 2mg11%

* Percent Daily Values are based on a 2000 calorie diet.

Slow Cooker Keto Pork Carnitas Bowls

Ingredients

- Carnitas
- 2 pounds pork
- 1/4 cup fresh orange juice
- 2 tbs olive oil
- 2 tbs tomato paste
- 2 tbs lime juice
- 2 tbs Coconut Aminos
- 1 tsp cumin
- 1 tsp Sea Salt

- 1/2 tsp Chili Powder

- 1/2 tsp oregano

- Cauliflower Rice

- 1 large head cauliflower

- 1/2 tbs olive oil

- 1/4 tsp cumin

- 1 tbs lime juice

- Sea Salt

Toppings

- 2 cups baby greens

- 1 cup Cherry Tomatoes

- 1/2 cup black olives

- 1/2 cup cheddar cheese

- salsa optional

- jalapenos optional

Instructions

1. Heat a skillet over high heat, and add olive oil. Quickly sear the outside of the pork roast.

2. In a small bowl, add the rest of the carnitas ingredients, and mix well.

3. Add the browned pork and the citrus marinade to the slow cooker. Cook on low for 3-4 hours.

4. When the pork is done, remove from the slow cooker, and shred with 2 forks. Return the pork to the slow cooker to soak up the marinade.

5. To prepare the cauliflower "rice," chop the cauliflower into small pieces, and then add to a food processor bowl. Process the cauliflower until it is in rice sized pieces. Be sure not to overprocess the cauliflower or it will get mushy while cooking.

6. The key to making fluffy and not watery cauliflower rice is to cook it over very high heat, and to only cook it for a few minutes, so the moisture doesn't begin to come out of it.

7. Use a large frying pan with 1 tablespoon olive oil. If using a smaller pan, cook the cauliflower rice in batches. Season with sea salt, cumin, and lime juice.

8. Top the cauliflower rice with shredded pork, and the rest of the toppings.

Macros for 1 out of 6 servings (without optional toppings)

41g Protein || 11g Carbs || 38g Fat || 554 Calories

Nutrition

Serving: 1meal | Calories: 554kcal | Carbohydrates: 11g | Protein: 41g | Fat: 38g

Slow-Cooker Garlic-Herb Mashed Cauliflower

INGREDIENTS

- 1 head cauliflower, cut into bite-size pieces
- 5 garlic cloves, smashed and peeled
- 4 cups vegetable broth
- 3 tablespoons butter, cut into cubes
- ⅓ cup Greek yogurt

- 2 tablespoons chopped fresh chives

- 1 tablespoon chopped fresh parsley

- 1 tablespoon chopped fresh rosemary

- 1 teaspoon garlic powder

- Salt and freshly ground black pepper

DIRECTIONS

Prep Time: 10 min | Cook Time: 3 hr

1. Place the cauliflower, garlic and broth inside the slow cooker. The cauliflower should be fully covered with broth. If it isn't (it can vary based on the size and shape of your slow cooker), add a little water until it is.

2. Turn the slow cooker on high and cook until the cauliflower is very tender, 2½ to 3 hours. Drain the cauliflower and garlic through a strainer, reserving ½ cup of the broth.

3. Use a potato masher or large fork to coarsely mash the cauliflower. Once it's coarsely mashed, add the butter and

yogurt, and mash until relatively smooth (if it's too stiff, ladle in up to ½ cup of the reserved cooking broth).

4. Stir in the chives, parsley, rosemary and garlic powder. Season with salt and pepper. Serve warm.

Crockpot Sausage And Peppers
RECIPE TIPS AND TRICKS:

If you use Spicy Sausage, you may want to cut back the crushed red pepper flakes just a bit and add more in at the end if you need to.

I used all Green Bell Peppers but any combination of colors would work here!

Note that if you leave the sausage in the slow cooker for too long, it can really lose its texture and become very soft. This doesn't bother me for a dish like this, but if the texture is a thing for you, keep this in mind.

INGREDIENTS

- 6 medium cloves garlic finely chopped
- 2 large yellow onions halved and thinly sliced
- 4 medium green bell peppers halved from top to bottom, cleaned and thinly sliced
- 1 Tablespoon kosher salt
- 1 teaspoon Italian Seasoning
- 1/4 teaspoon dried oregano
- 1/2 teaspoon crushed red pepper flakes
- 28 ounces canned unsalted crushed tomatoes
- 1/4 cup cold water
- 1 bay leaf
- 2 pounds uncooked Italian Sausage Links (approx 6 to 8 sausages)) Mild or Spicy
- chopped Italian parsley for serving optional

INSTRUCTIONS

1. Finely chop garlic. I used my food processor with the chopping blade to save time.

2. If you are using a food processor, swap the chopping blade for the slicing disc. Peel onions and halve. Place the onion halves cut side down in the food processor and slice. Alternately, thinly slice by hand. Remove the chopped garlic and sliced onion and place into the slow cooker insert.

3. Slice bell peppers in half from top to bottom. Remove the ribs and any seeds.

4. Proceed to thinly slice or use the food processor to slice exactly like the onions.

5. Add the sliced bell peppers to the slow cooker along with the salt, Italian Seasoning, dried oregano, crushed red pepper flakes, 1/4 cup cold water and can of crushed tomatoes. Toss until well coated and liquid is evenly distributed.

6. Remove about half of the peppers and onion mixture to a bowl. Bury the uncooked sausages in the middle and return the peppers and onions back to the slow cooker to cover the sausage. Add the bay leaf.

7. Cover, set to low and cook for 6 hours. The onions and peppers will give off a lot of water as they cook which will make the sauce liquid and spoon-able so don't stress that there isn't enough liquid.

8. Top with some chopped parsley, serve hot and Enjoy!

Slow Cooker Low Carb Zuppa Toscana Soup (Keto-Friendly)

Ingredients

- 1 lb mild or hot ground Italian sausage
- 1 tbsp oil
- ½ cup finely diced onion or 1 medium onion
- 3 garlic cloves, minced
- 36 oz chicken or vegetable stock
- 1 large cauliflower head, diced into small florets
- 3 cups chopped kale
- ¼ tsp crushed red pepper flakes
- 1 tsp salt
- ½ tsp pepper

- ½ cup heavy cream

Instructions

1. Brown the ground sausage in a skillet over medium heat until done.
2. Using a slotted spoon, remove the sausage and place it into at least a 6-quart slow cooker. Discard the grease.
3. Place the oil in the same skillet and saute the onions for 3-4 minutes or until translucent.
4. Add the onions, chicken or vegetable stock, cauliflower florets, kale, crushed red pepper flakes, salt, and pepper to the slow cooker. Mix until combined.
5. Cook on high for 4 hours or on low for 8 hours.
6. Add the heavy cream and mix until combined.

Easy Tomato Basil Soup (Instant Pot and Slow Cooker Soup)

Ingredients

- Tomato and Basil Soup
- 3 tbsp butter
- 3 tbsp olive oil
- 1 medium onion, diced
- 2 ribs celery, diced
- 2 garlic cloves, minced
    - 1/2 cups fresh basil, diced (or 1/4 cup dried)
- 1 tbsp fresh oregano, diced (or 1 tsp dried)
- 1 bay leaf
- 2 tbsp tomato paste
- (2) 28 oz can whole or diced tomatoes (or 3 to 4 lbs fresh tomatoes, peeled and seeded. Cut into chunks)
- 1-1/2 cups vegetable broth
- 1 tbsp white wine vinegar (balsamic vinegar is a great option too!)
- 1 tsp salt
- 1/2 tsp pepper

- 1-1/2 cups parmesan cheese grated

- 1/2 cup whipping cream

- Parmesan Cheese Crisps (Optional)

- 6 tbsp parmesan cheese, grated

- 3 tsp. fresh basil

- sprinkle of garlic powder

Instructions

1. Pressure cooker method:

2. Select Saute setting, medium heat. Add olive oil and butter and melt. Add onions and celery and cook until soft. Add garlic and cook 1 minute. Add basil, oregano, bay leaf, tomato paste, tomatoes, vegetable broth, white wine vinegar, salt, and pepper to the pot. Secure the lid and pressure cook on High for 4 minutes.

3. Once cooking is complete, allow the pot to release pressure naturally for 10 minutes, then do a quick release. Remove lid carefully. Remove bay leaf, then

using an immersion blender directly in the pressure cooker, blend soup until desired consistency is reached. Alternatively, you can process smaller portions in a blender and add back into the pot in batches.

4. In a small bowl add 1/2 cup of hot soup and mix with whipping cream. Add into the pot. Add parmesan cheese. Select Sauté, medium heat, and warm until cheese is melted and soup is desired temperature, stirring frequently.

Stovetop method:

1. In a skillet, over medium-high heat on melt butter and olive oil. Sauté onions and celery until soft. Add garlic and cook 1 minute. Add basil, oregano, bay leaf, tomato paste, tomatoes, vegetable broth, white wine vinegar, salt, and pepper to the pot. Bring to a boil, cover and simmer for 30 minutes.

2. Remove bay leaf, then using an immersion blender directly in the pot, blend soup until desired consistency is reached. Alternatively, you can process smaller portions in a blender and add back into the pot in batches.

3. In a small bowl add 1/2 cup of hot soup and mix with whipping cream. Add into the pot. Add parmesan cheese. Over medium heat, melt the cheese and warm soup until the desired temperature is reached, stirring frequently

Slow Cooker method:

1. In a skillet, over medium-high heat on melt butter and olive oil. Sauté onions and celery until soft. Add garlic and cook 1 minute. Add basil, oregano, bay leaf, tomato paste, tomatoes, vegetable broth, white wine vinegar, salt, and pepper to the pot. Cover and cook on Low for 6 to 8 hours.

2. Remove bay leaf, then using an immersion blender directly in the slow cooker, blend soup until desired consistency is reached. Alternatively, you can process smaller portions in a blender and add back into the pot in batches.

3. In a small bowl add 1/2 cup of hot juices and mix with whipping cream. Add into the pot. Add parmesan cheese. Continue to melt the cheese and warm soup until the desired temperature is reached, stirring occasionally.

Parmesan Cheese Crisp Recipe:

1. Preheat oven to 350 degrees F. On a cookie sheet with a piece of parchment paper, drop 1 tbsp of parmesan for each crisp. Top with fresh basil and a sprinkle of garlic powder. Spread out evenly. Bake 10 to 15 minutes until golden and crispy.

To Serve:

- Garnish with a little whipping cream, a sprinkle of cheese and basil and a delicious parmesan crisp! Adjust seasoning, salt, and pepper as needed!

Notes

Dried basil makes a great substitution but I've found the taste of dried basil varies. Start with 1/4 cup and add more until the taste is to your liking.

Blend the soup to your desired thickness. Some people love it chunky (like me), others like it smooth.

Instant Pot Garlic Parmesan Chicken

A few notes about the ingredients:

Chicken: I used chicken breasts but you can also use chicken thighs or bone-in chicken. The cooking time will be a little different, just check the notes section in the recipe below.

Half and half: if you don't have any half and half you can use half milk and half cream or you can use evaporated milk.

Flour: I used flour to thicken my sauce but if you want to make this recipe gluten free you can also use a cornstarch slurry.

Parmesan cheese: I use parmesan cheese that I buy in a big bag from Costco, it's pre-grated. It worked well for this garlic parmesan chicken. You can use parmesan cheese off the block and if you're in a pinch you can even use the stuff from the green can.

When cooking with pot in pot pasta: When I cook the pasta at the same time in the same pot I like to bump up the seasonings a bunch. I like to add in twice as much salt, pepper, garlic powder, garlic and parmesan cheese. If not, the dish will be pretty bland. Always season to taste at the end of the cooking time as well!

INGREDIENTS

- 2 Tbsp butter

- 1 small yellow onion, diced

- 4 large garlic cloves, minced

- 1/2 cup chicken broth

- 1/2 tsp garlic powder

- 1/4 tsp pepper

- 1/2 tsp salt

- 8 oz sliced mushrooms (optional)

- 1 1/2 lbs boneless skinless breasts sliced into 1/2 inch filets

- 1 cup half and half

- 2 Tbsp flour

- 1/2 cup parmesan cheese

- 3 oz coarsely chopped spinach

- Salt and freshly ground pepper

To make with pasta:

- 10 ounces uncooked fettuccine noodles or linguine noodles

- 3 cups water

2. Turn your Instant Pot to the saute setting (more). When the display reads HOT add in the butter. Once the butter is melted add in the onions and saute for about 3-4 minutes. Add in the garlic and saute for 30 seconds. Add in the chicken broth, garlic powder, pepper and salt. Stir. Add in the mushrooms (if using) and chicken.

3. Optional: If you want to cook pasta at the same time and in the same pot you can. Just get a pan that will fit inside your Instant Pot* and fill it with 3 cups or water and then break 10 ounces of fettuccine or linguine noodles to fit inside the pan (see my note below). Carefully place the pan on top of the chicken. I use a homemade silicone sling that I cut from a silicone baking mat* to lower my pan down onto the chicken. You can also make a foil sling.

4. Cover the pot and secure the lid. Make sure valve is set to sealing. Set the manual/pressure cook button to

6 minutes (this is the cooking time for the 1/2 inch pieces of chicken breast, if they are thicker than that you may need more time). Let the pressure release naturally for 10 minutes and then move the valve to "venting."

5. Remove the lid. If you are cooking pasta, carefully remove the pan of pasta and set aside. Use tongs to place the chicken on a platter. Loosely cover with foil. Turn the Instant Pot to the saute setting. Warm the half and half up in a pyrex measuring cup for 45 seconds in the microwave. Whisk the flour into the half and half until it's smooth. Whisk the mixture into the Instant Pot. This will thicken up the sauce in a few minutes. Add in the parmesan cheese. Add in the spinach. Salt and pepper to taste. If using pasta, drain any water off of the pasta and stir into the pot.

6. Serve sauce (and optional pasta) with the chicken.

Crock Pot Fire Roasted Tomato Shrimp Tacos

You'll love this shrimp taco recipe because it's made in a slow cooker. Crock Pot tacos require SO little prep! Slow cooking the shrimp with fire roasted tomatoes (and other vegetables) produces delicious flavor and preserves nutrients!

INGREDIENTS

- 1 lb medium shrimp, peeled and tails off (fresh or frozen then thawed) (see notes below for fresh shrimp)
- 1 tbsp olive oil (or avocado oil)
- 1/2 cup chopped onion
- 14.5 oz can fire roasted stewed tomatoes (diced work best)
- 1/2 cup chunky salsa
- 1 bell pepper, chopped (about 1/2 to 2/3 cup)
- dash of sea salt and black pepper
- 1/2 tsp cumin
- 1/2 tsp chili powder or ancho chili powder (see notes for substitutes)

- 1/4 tsp paprika or cayenne pepper
  - o tsp minced garlic
- 3–4 tbsp chopped cilantro (2 –3 tbsp for plating)

Optional toppings – extra chopped green onion, sour cream, avocado, jalapeno pepper, etc.

Tortillas to serve (gluten free corn, paleo tortillas or gluten free flour tortillas)

INSTRUCTIONS

1. First make sure your shrimp are peeled and tails off. If you are using frozen shrimp, quickly thaw in water for 10 minutes, then peel.
2. Layer your raw shrimp at the bottom of pot. Drizzle with 1 tbsp olive oil. Then mix in your chopped onion.
3. Drain your canned fire roasted tomatoes and then pour it over the shrimp. Stir together.

4. Add your bell pepper and the rest of your ingredients, including your seasonings and cilantro. Stir all together.

5. Place slow cooker (crock pot) low for 2-3 hrs. Or high for 90 minutes to 2 hours.

6. Check on shrimp around 1 hour of cooking on high. If they look almost done, place on medium for another 30 minutes to hour. They should be seasoned nicely and pink, similar to that of steamed shrimp.

7. Serve with gluten free corn or paleo tortillas, chopped cabbage/salad, rice, or avocado!

8. Top with extra cilantro and jalapeno and gluten free flour tortillas

Paleo Pork Roast Slow Cooker Recipe with Chimichurri Sauce

INGREDIENTS

- 2–3 Pound Pork Roast (boneless)
- 4 Tbl Extra Virgin Olive Oil (divided)

    o Pound Carrots (trimmed and quartered lengthwise)

- 1 Sweet Onion (thickly sliced)
- Real Salt * (to taste)
- 1 Recipe chimichurri sauce

INSTRUCTIONS

1. Place the pork roast in a crock pot. Drizzle 2 tablespoons of the olive oil over the roast and sprinkle it with salt and pepper. Cover with the lid and cook it on high for 6 hours (or low for 12 hours).

2. After the roast has been in the crock pot for 4 hours (8 hours on low), add the onions and carrots to the crock pot, placing around the roast (Alternatively, you can pan fry the onions and carrots with the remaining 2 tablespoons of olive oil and saute them on medium/high heat until they begin to caramelize. Add them to the crock pot after this step).

3. Cook the roast, carrots, and onions for 2 more hours (4 hours on low), or until the pork is pulls apart easily and carrots are soft.

4. Place the roast, carrots, and onions on a serving platter and drizzle with chimichurri sauce. Serve with extra sauce.

Keto Low Carb Chili Recipe - Crock Pot Or Instant Pot (Paleo)

INGREDIENTS

- 2 1/2 lbGround beef
- 1/2 large Onion (chopped)
- 8 cloves Garlic (minced)
- 2 15-oz canDiced tomatoes (with liquid)
    - 6-oz canTomato paste
- 1 4-oz canGreen chiles (with liquid)
    - tbspWorcestershire sauce
- 1/4 cupChili powder
    - tbspCumin

- 1 tbspDried oregano

- 2 tspSea salt

- 1 tspBlack pepper

- 1 mediumBay leaf (optional)

INSTRUCTIONS

1. Crock Pot slow cooker instructions

2. In a skillet over medium-high heat, cook the chopped onion for 5-7 minutes, until translucent (or increase the time to about 20 minutes if you like them caramelized). Add the garlic and cook for a minute or less, until fragrant.

3. Add the ground beef. Cook for 8-10 minutes, breaking apart with a spatula, until browned.

4. Transfer the ground beef mixture into a slow cooker. Add remaining ingredients, except bay leaf, and stir until combined. Place the bay leaf into the middle, if using.

5. Cook for 6-8 hours on low or 3-4 hours on high. If you
    used a bay leaf, remove it before serving.

Instant Pot pressure cooker instructions

1. Select the "Sauté" setting on the pressure cooker (this
    part is done without the lid). Add the chopped onion
    and cook for 5-7 minutes, until translucent (or increase
    the time to about 20 minutes if you like them
    caramelized). Add the garlic and cook for a minute or
    less, until fragrant.
2. Add the ground beef. Cook for 8-10 minutes, breaking
    apart with a spatula, until browned.
3. Add remaining ingredients, except bay leaf, to the
    Instant Pot and stir until combined. (For the Instant
    Pot version, it is recommended to also add a cup of
    water or broth.) Place the bay leaf into the middle, if
    using.

4. Close the lid. Press "Keep Warm/Cancel" to stop the saute cycle. Select the "Meat/Stew" setting (35 minutes) to start pressure cooking.

5. Wait for the natural release if you can, or turn the valve to "vent" for quick release if you're short on time. If you used a bay leaf, remove it before serving.

Gumbo Meal Prep

Ingredients

- 1/4 cup olive oil
- 4 cloves garlic minced
  - medium onion chopped
  - tsp thyme
- 1 tsp Salt
- 1/4 tsp cayenne pepper
  - cups chicken broth
- 1 lb boneless chicken thighs cubed
  - andouille sausages
- 1 can diced tomatoes

- 2 tbs tomato paste

- 2 cups okra sliced

- 2 medium bell peppers diced

- 2 cups riced cauliflower

Instructions

1. In a skillet, brown sausages. Remove to slice.

2. In the same skillet, add olive oil, garlic, onions, salt, and spices. Saute until lightly browned. Add the sliced sausages back in the pan with the onions.

3. In a crockpot, add the rest of the ingredients, and then add the sauteed onions and sausages. Slow cook on low for 4-5 hours, or on high for 2-3 hours, until all vegetables are tender.

4. This spicy stew freezes well for up to 3 months in an airtight container.

Nutrition for 1 out of 6 servings (including provolone and avocado)

26.1g Protein | 18.1g Carbs | 35.6g Fat | 8.3g Fiber | 501 Calories

Notes: If your fat needs are higher than 70%, thicken with coconut milk. Rather than using a Roux as traditional with Gumbo, this one relies on tomatoes and okra, so leaving out the okra will make a thinner stew.